T0095192

# TRAVEL THE WORLD

## and never get sick again

# TRAVEL THE WORLD
## and never get sick again
### "Natural Therapies For Prevention"

## Dr. Fadairo Afolabi

CEO and Founder of The Reverend Eugene and Mary
Robinson Center For Wellness and Longevity

iUniverse, Inc.
Bloomington

Travel The World And Never Get Sick Again
"Natural Therapies For Prevention"

Copyright © 2010 by Dr. Fadairo Afolabi

All rights reserved. No part of this book may be used or reproduced by any means, graphic, electronic, or mechanical, including photocopying, recording, taping or by any information storage retrieval system without the written permission of the publisher except in the case of brief quotations embodied in critical articles and reviews.

iUniverse books may be ordered through booksellers or by contacting:

iUniverse
1663 Liberty Drive
Bloomington, IN 47403
www.iuniverse.com
1-800-Authors (1-800-288-4677)

Because of the dynamic nature of the Internet, any Web addresses or links contained in this book may have changed since publication and may no longer be valid. The views expressed in this work are solely those of the author and do not necessarily reflect the views of the publisher, and the publisher hereby disclaims any responsibility for them.

ISBN: 978-1-4502-7184-4 (sc)
ISBN: 978-1-4502-7186-8 (ebk)

Printed in the United States of America

iUniverse rev. date: 12/08/2010

# DEDICATION

This book is affectionately dedicated to the following people. To my late parents, Reverend Eugene and Mary Robinson, who taught me the appreciation of travel and exploration. Mommy and Daddy were my first travel agents who wanted their children to explore boundaries beyond their own while staying healthy in the process. They were holistic advocates who believed in the innate power of the body, mind and spirit to heal it self when given proper nutrition, exercise and positive thinking.

My parents paved the way for me to not only share this information with my readers and patients, but also to establish the REVEREND EUGENE & MARY ROBINSON CENTER FOR WELLNESS AND LONGEVITY, a center for holistic and natural therapies. For them, I continue their legacy through my work with family, friends and patients.

To my husband, Earl, a wonderful travel partner who also enjoys the art and science of travel.

To my outstanding, distinguished and loving children, Jubba, Fashade, Sobande, and Sosanya, who were exposed to my passion for travel early in life. To my grandson, Zakai, who will travel beyond his creative imagination. Special thanks to Sobande, who worked tirelessly with me in preparation for this book. You have all been my rock, and source of great encouragement, strength and support in all my endeavors. I know you will continue to explore God's Green Earth with passion and desire. May this book be your guide to staying healthy on your spiritual and earthly journey.

# ACKNOWLEGEMENTS

I thank God, the navigator of my life, from whom all blessings flow.

I would also like to thank my travel partners, Jamillah and Yasin Muhammadi, Patrice Johnson, James Alonzo, Cynthia and Ron Harris, Patricia Howard, Iman Hamilton and Florence Mason, for helping to make my travel experiences stimulating, exciting and inspirational.

Special thanks to my editor and dear friend, Mrs. Ricki Stevenson, who has been my sounding board for this book.

Sincere thanks to my best friend and spiritual advisor, Annie Pauline Pierce, for your love and enthusiastic support for over 50 years.

To my big sis, Georgette Addison, thanks for your unconditional love and support.

And to my colleague and unconditional loving friend, who has always "had my back", Dr. Michelle Cox Spivey, thank you for your inspiring words, your love of life, positivity, enthusiasm, and faith in me. I salute you.

And finally to my long term Golden friends, Kathie Osborne, Amelia "Niki" Gamble, Cleta McLeod and Faye Wiggins, thank you for your many years of support, love and camaraderie.

# CONTENTS

Introduction . . . . . . . . . . . . . . . . . . . . . . . . . . . . . . . . . . . 1

Chapter 1    Travel the World and Never Get Sick Again . . . . 7

Chapter 2    Your Overall Health . . . . . . . . . . . . . . . . . . . . 15

Chapter 3    The Immune System . . . . . . . . . . . . . . . . . . . 25

Chapter 4    Colon Health . . . . . . . . . . . . . . . . . . . . . . . . . 35

Chapter 5    Preparation . . . . . . . . . . . . . . . . . . . . . . . . . . 39

Chapter 6    Spiritual Health. . . . . . . . . . . . . . . . . . . . . . . 57

Chapter 7    On Your Return . . . . . . . . . . . . . . . . . . . . . . 61

Chapter 8    Conclusion . . . . . . . . . . . . . . . . . . . . . . . . . . 67

# INTRODUCTION

⌒⁄⁄⌒

## By Ricki Stevenson

I am a woman of many passions, but I am most passionate about traveling the world, meeting new and interesting people, being introduced to different nationalities, history and customs, lifting up the edge of the rug, so to speak, to peak into the deeper aspects of various cultures and partaking of the foods of those cultures.

As a little girl my parents exposed me to every kind of food, neighborhood and culture available! Looking back, I realize some kids might not have fond memories of their parents taking them south of the border to Tijuana, for the obligatory sombrero-on-the head, seated-on-the-painted-donkey photo. But to this day, I remember with mouth watering clarity, the hot Mexican carrots and chilies that came with the tacos, daddy bought on the street. So delicious, and different from the tacos mom made at home.

Forget that eggs, milk and orange juice, foods my parents forced fed us (to build strong bones) for breakfast that made me violently sick to the stomach. I learned early on that certain foods I dare not eat, or wind up tied to the toilet for days.

Summer trips to great grandfather's farm in Milo, Oklahoma were jammed packed with down home soul food that my Denver-raised mother rarely served. Everything we ate was home grown, raised, killed, smoked and cooked right there at home. Breakfast at grandma's house might include fried fish, fried chicken, smoked ham and bacon, biscuits, collard greens from the yard, milk from the cow in the barn and the eggs collected from the chicken coop. Strange, I don't remember ever getting sick.

Fast forward to my first international forays into the world of culture and cuisine. A post grad trip to Jamaica and Haiti introduced me to fascinating new foods and tastes that linger in my mind and mouth to this day!

Parrot fish with onions, jerk chicken, ackee and salt fish, beef patties, goat curry, coco bread with slabs of yellow cheese, mangoes, pineapples and bananas bought at the outdoor market, flavored slushies (wid da condensed sweet cream, ) and coconut ice cream. Many of these delicacies bought on the street or at roadside stops. I'm drinking the water, drinking the Ting (a carbonated grapefruit soft drink) drinking the home made ginger beer and NEVER ONCE did I get sick. However one year later, a trip to Mazatlan proved disastrous. Two days into our Mexican getaway, after a shrimp taco lunch on the beach, a bottled soft drink, bottled water and an ice cream cone bought on the street, I wanted to die! Between throwing up and getting up (to go to the toilet) I lost 8 pounds and couldn't wait to get back home. I was determined this would never happen again. No more eating off the mean streets for me! I became the cautious traveler. No ice in my drinks, no home made drinks, no ice cream from street vendors, I brushed my teeth with bottled water and ate no fruits or veggies that weren't cooked or washed off with bottled water. It was challenging, but the caution worked.

This caution carried me safely through gastronomic trips to Rome, Florence, Venice and Capri, Italy; a stay in Damman, Saudi Arabia where the seafood was enormous, plentiful and inexpensive and for me always cooked, and where we had to go fetch desalinized water several times a week. A trip to Hong Kong, where we followed the Saturday lunch crowds to the largest dum sum restaurant I've seen in life. A football-size dining experience that lasted three hours and included cooked foods I'd never even thought of eating. A trip to Trinidad for Carnival that featured the tastiest traditional cuisine; return trips to Jamaica and Haiti (piece of cake); an array of pan-Asian foods in Hawaii and nectar of the Gods, fresh picked-from-the-field "sugar baby" pineapples from the island of Lanai; and a successful return trip to Mexico (Cancun this time) where I was oh-so-careful that I don't remember what I ate or drank, but I didn't get sick. I wavered only once, during a trip to Grenada. I hesitated when an elder woman approached me on the beach selling homemade chocolates from a basket on her head. My desire overcame my caution though and I tasted the most amazingly pure chocolate confection I've ever tasted, a taste I still dream of.

I was totally caught off guard in 1990, when on assignment as a television travel reporter in Glasgow, Scotland, I came down with a horrible case of MacDougal's Revenge. I blamed the haggis (a traditional Scottish breakfast dish), but the doctor said it may have been the water I used while brushing my teeth. (okay...so I let my guard down there.) I was cautious again when I moved to Paris, France in 1997 with my then eleven year old daughter. We started out drinking bottled water. With so many to choose from (with gas, without gas, with extra bubbles, with extra minerals) it took a few months before we hit upon a brand with a taste worthy of being called "Oakland Water" (my home town). But soon we were drinking water straight from the tap. Interestingly, I have had guests and clients ask me about the safety of eating in Parisian restaurants. Never in twelve years have I heard of anyone who has gotten sick after a dining experience in the City of Light. Based on these experiences, you can imagine it was of great interest to me when I met Dr. Fa, as she is affectionately known by her patients, in May, 2008. She and her husband, Earl, were visiting Paris with a group of well heeled, seasoned travelers, who had been making trips to Africa, the Caribbean, and around the world for years. Their goal (and my challenge) was to help them to cover as much physical and cultural ground as possible, while squeezing maximum value out of the weakened US dollar. I'd learned the greatest experiences aren't always based on how much money you spend, but on how much of yourself you are willing to invest into an experience. Dr. Fa shared my enthusiasm and zeal in this regard and we immediately hit it off, based on her spirit of going with the flow and looking forward to the possibilities, plus she talked about how to travel the world, eat and not get sick.

As the group moved through our days together in Paris, Dr. Fa was excited and knowledgeable about the African and African American history I shared. She kept pace as we strolled the Champs Elysees or rue de la Goutte D'Or in Little Africa. She quickly picked up on the French cultural cues: greeting bus drivers and vendors with "Bonjour Monsieur/Madame", and did not get upset when the restaurant service was slow; or the food wasn't just like home. She was my kind of world traveler! During the last two years I've gotten to know more about Dr. Fa, the professional holistic Chiropractic Physician, community health advisor and natural healer. I've attended fascinating seminars at the Robinson Wellness Center, in East Orange, New Jersey. I have listened to her lectures and heard her speak on many occasions of how to care for our bodies, how to eat to live and not live to eat, how to keep the weight off, and how to keep the mind and body and spirit uplifted to maximize our time and enjoyment on earth. I urge you to read her book and put her ideas to use. It's up to you to live your best life!

Ricki Stevenson
Founder/CEO, Black Paris Tours

# CHAPTER 1

*✼*

# TRAVEL THE WORLD AND NEVER GET SICK AGAIN.

## "Natural Therapies For Prevention"

*"We shall not seek from exploration*
*And the end of all our exploring*
*Will be to arrive where we started*
*And know the place for the first time."*
*T.S. Elliot*

If you have traveled outside the United States you probably have experienced the, "Oh so" dreaded "Montezuma's Revenge". The term originated in Mexico where unsuspecting travelers have drank the water or have eaten food tainted with bacteria. If you are not familiar with this term it simply means that you have been infected, with a bacteria known as "Escherichia Coli," otherwise known as "E Coli", and in many cases called "Traveler's Diarrhea" or "TD"

I begin my story with Montezuma's Revenge because travelers are most familiar with its consequences. E Coli is a bacterium that enters your system as a foreign entity disturbing the natural order or your bodily functions. It originates from food, water, person - person contact and unclean environments. Some travelers become severely ill, experiencing diarrhea, vomiting, stomach pain, abdominal cramps, nausea, bloating, lower back and neck pain and severe headaches. These symptoms have also been attributed to a change in environment, change in eating habits, change in bowel function, and change in the types of food you are accustomed to, ice served in drinks, water from brushing your teeth, gargling and a change in local environmental influences. E Coli will ruin any of your travel plans, and you will find yourself devoid of the pleasure and excitement you expected to have on your trip.

I recall my first trip to West Africa. I traveled with a small group of men and women to Accra, Ghana. It was 1996 and my second time traveling abroad. It was a small but bustling town, with lots of people going about their normal day. It was a colorful sight, as the men and women adorned in their traditional African garb and speaking in their native tongues, went about their day. The atmosphere had a powerful, but not offensive, earthy smell as well as the aroma emanating from the roadside grills, as the vendors cooked their traditional cuisines. It was my first time in West Africa, and quite a different and unique experience. Much different than East Africa, where I had spent a month and a half, back packing through Kenya and Tanzania. In East Africa, the customs and traditional garb there were not everyday wear. As a matter of fact, European clothes were seen more often as the everyday wear in that part of Africa. As we traveled to our hotel by bus, I peered from the window to get a glance of the strange looking food smoking on the many homemade grills we passed. I wasn't familiar with what I saw and every vendor we passed had this strange meat on their grill. It resembled a large rat or medium sized possum. I found out from our driver, it was called "akrantie", the "grasscutter" and it was a very popular meat among the locals. Its main function and purpose is to eat grass, hence the name, but the locals found this meat to be quite tasty. We had a wonderful time in Ghana, discovering much of our history, visiting the Elmina Castle and conversing with the many Americans who live in the surrounding area. Most of the food in the hotels was quite tasty and they catered to many tourists, having a menu of familiar dishes and European cuisine.

We were escorted to many surrounding cities, places of interests and traditional African villages by Mama Dokono, the Oprah Winfrey of Accra. She is an actress in a Ghanaian soap opera, the host of a children's program called "Fireside Chat", and a good friend of one of our travelers. She was known all over Ghana and privy to places common tourists would not be allowed. Because of her, we were able to visit the palace of the Ashanti tribesmen and meet their King and his entourage. Our visit there was very revealing as we learned the history of the very proud Ashanti people.

The trip was going well until we went on an outing to the beach.

The story is as follows.

We relaxed at a table and chairs that were set up on the beach and enjoyed the heat of the day, the warm ocean water and the intriguing stories and conversations on world issues we shared with one another. We had not been there long when a gentleman approached our table, dressed in a waiters or cooks white uniform, and asked if we would like something to eat from the beach restaurant. He handed us menus and waited for our response. The menu looked very enticing and I decided to order the fish with rice and beans. After all this was a good place to eat fresh fish, this was a fishing town.

Everyone placed their orders. All decided to stick with familiar foods, some ordered chicken and others ordered the same fish I did. When the meals arrived, everything appeared in order. We partook, and enjoyed the meal with smiles and laughter. We then rode horses on the beach, took a myriad of photos, splashed around in the ocean water and bathed in the sun until the day was over. As the sun went down, we packed up our things and returned to the hotel. The day had come to an end. We were all tired, but satisfied with our days' experiences. We headed to bed.

The next day, I awoke early feeling nauseous with a terrible stomach pain. The pain was a burning, indescribable fire in my belly. I rushed into the bathroom, where every orifice of my body had something trying to escape. I was "sick as a dog". I went to lie back down on the bed, when I heard a knock on my door and a voice saying, "are you ready? We will be ready to go in about 15 minutes". I knew right then, I couldn't possibly go anywhere. I was so sick, it was frightening. I thought I might have to go to the hospital. But I decided to endure and wait it out. I stayed in my room all day, going back and forth to the bathroom, emptying my bowels in every way my body would allow. I found out later that evening that everyone who ate the same fish I did yesterday was sick as well.

I returned back to that beach several days later to discover the obvious. The restaurant was a small wooden structure with a large open air grill. The structure had a partial roof protected its contents from the rain. Heavy transparent plastic was rolled up on each side attached to the edging, apparently to close off the open sides when it rains. On the grill were all types of meat mixed together-some cooked and some cooking. Chicken, fish, beef, and akrantie, sizzling on the grill, a few inches apart from one another. To the naked eye, the restaurant appeared clean enough, despite the flies, but I believe to this day, that my American gastric system was not use to the traditional, authentic, Ghanaian home cooking, with their wonderful blend of ingredients, special herbs and spices. I didn't have a clue as to how long the fish was exposed to the elements, or even if the fish was fresh or how sanitary the grill and counter tops were. These conditions were sure contributors to foreign bacteria and to what made those of us who ate the fish, very sick a few days before.

Ever since my trip to Ghana, and that frightening experience, I have traveled all over the world to major cities, rural environments and third world countries. I have eaten indigenous foods, drank their libations, eaten their wild life and local herbs and have never gotten sick. I attribute my success to a few simple techniques: learn as much as you can about the country, its food, its attractions, its traditions, tours and environment. Many countries outside the United States have their own unique identity, specific energy, customs and local protocols: protocols for eating, family traditions and maybe even attire, which may include the color and length of a garment. These protocols may even be required for specific times of day and specific festivals and or functions.

Always be respectful and aware of the cultural differences in order not to offend. Pay attention to any instructions given to you by a guide if you have one; become in tune or at one with your environment-spiritually and physically.

Physically meaning, be vigilante, cautious and aware of your surroundings at all times. Be aware of your space as well as the personal space of others.

Spiritually, meaning, you will reap the benefits manifested by your positive thoughts and actions. Expand your mind, let go of any restrictions, judgments and fears: let the experience come to you. You will begin to sense and feel part of the world. You will learn to appreciate and understand differences in people, their culture, religion and their way of life.

Travel with love, and love fiercely. Surrender to joy and be enchanted by its treasures. Surrender to wellness and stay positive as you explore a brand new exhilarating adventure. Your spirit, your emotions and physical well being are paramount to your good health. They arc all connected and apart of what makes you the person you are. When one is out of balance they are all affected. Homeostasis is the balance of this trilogy of optimum health. All three must be fed with the fuels that keep them vibrant and alive. Love, being the main dish or fuel.

The spirit is fed love, grace, forgiveness and positive thought. Your emotions are fed with love, peace, tranquility, kindness, brotherhood and prayer. Your physical body is fed with love, good nutrition, touch and exercise.

By following a few simple steps in preparation for your trip, you, too, can travel and never get sick. These steps are outlined for you in Chapter 6.

# CHAPTER 2

Your Overall Health

Your health is your wealth. Let me say that again – Your health is your wealth. Your health is the most important aspect to your total well being. When we are sick, our bodies take us through an emotional rollercoaster. We feel spiritually, physically and emotionally depleted. Our bodies are stressed to the point where we may experience aches and pains, discomfort and many sleepless nights.

The key to avoid these symptoms is to create a balanced environment in the body called "homeostasis". It is your innate intelligence, your natural given healing ability, to bring the body to its optimal level. Our bodies are little miracles wonderfully made to correct and heal themselves if given a positive, healthy and balanced environment.

Our bodies react to all things that we consume. It takes in what it needs and eliminates what it doesn't need. These are the things to which we need to pay much attention. Many of our illnesses come from improper elimination leading to impacted colons. Toxins from these impactions build up in our bodies and run havoc through our system causing sickness and disease.

What we put in our bodies must be eliminated frequently. We should be eliminating as many times a day as we consume food. Therefore if you eat three meals a day, you should be eliminating three times a day.

Further, without proper elimination, you may become sluggish and lack energy that is needed for a vibrant and fulfilling life. Conversely, if you are putting in nutritional, live foods, full of natural vitamins, minerals and enzymes, the body can absorb these and put them to work in the cells to revitalize you on a day to day basis. These enzymes, minerals and vitamins then act as a catalyst for daily elimination.

I know you have heard the expression "Garbage in Garbage Out".

Well, it's true. If you are putting into your body foods that have no nutritional value, then your body becomes void of nutrition, it then begins to break down at a faster rate, causing sickness, disease and eventually death.

In addition to maintaining optimal physical health, we also must maintain environmental, spiritual and emotional health.

We can become sick from our negative thoughts. We can become sick from negative environments. Our thoughts become manifest in the universe positively as well as negatively. There is tremendous power in words and thought. Always be ready to transform the negative into positive.

Therefore, we must always look to consume healthy foods, place ourselves in healthy environment and train our minds to maintain healthy emotional states. All of these things we need to keep us strong, vibrant, energetic and active, whether we are traveling or not.

So when traveling and you encounter some environmental abnormalities, putrid smells or unsightly encounters, and you will, just go with the flow, keep moving and don't let an imperfect experience turn you off or cause you to miss an important cultural or educational event. Stay positive, stay focused and be delighted to be involved in new cultural experiences. Here is a perfect example of how negative environments can affect your thoughts, attitudes and actions.

In 1972, I traveled from Kenya to Tanzania by local bus and WOW!, what an eye opener. I waited in the market square with a group of local tribesmen and women from the Massai and Kikuyu tribes. It was an extremely humid and sweltering day. I estimated the degrees in the high 90's. I was extremely thirsty, so I went into a small, un-painted, open air, wooden store to purchase a soda. I asked for a coke and to my surprise, I received a warm bottle of Coca Cola shaped like the bottles from back in the day, the ones with the waistlines. I wondered what ever happened to those bottles. I guess they were all shipped to Africa. I laughed to myself, and then suddenly realized that this coke wasn't cold. Did they not have refrigeration? This was my first eye opener. But I was not going to let that disturb my peace of mind on this very hot and humid day. After a few minutes of getting my Swahili together I was able to ask the merchant, "Do you have any cold Coca Cola."?

His response, "You didn't ask for a cold one, biridi sana, that's how you ask for a cold one," A new lesson learned and question answered. Yes, they did have refrigeration, but warm or cold you had a choice and you had to make that choice known.

After that experience, I filed away the terminology and never forgot how to say cold in Swahili again.

When the bus arrived, it was the size of a school bus and had a large luggage rack on top. People rushed over to load their luggage and belongings onto the rack and boarded with their children as well as their chickens. One passenger even had a goat. I hurried over to the bus and watched the mannerisms of the locals to observe the protocol.

I sat on the bus next to the indigenous Maasi, a Chief. He was dressed in all his cultural attire (a wrap around red cloth extending over his right shoulder), a hunting spear at his side, and his hair wrapped with red clay into a tight (what we would call today a "doobee". He had a large hole in his right ear lobe that housed a can of his chewing tobacco and wore several large beaded earrings in his left ear. The multi-colored circular beads around his neck were extremely beautiful and certainly outstanding. It was obvious in his mannerism, that he was of royal descent. The bus pulled off, and we were headed to Dar Es Salaam, Tanzania. This was just the beginning of an adventure of simplistic beauty and a journey of mysteries waiting to be revealed. I was ready- mentally, physically, spiritually and emotionally.

We moved along fairly well, even with the very rough unpaved rocky and narrow dirt roads. The bus bounced us from side to side, as we were seated two in a row. I was seated on the outside of the row and had to extend my neck a bit to take in the view from the window. I felt the Chief's spear hit the side of my right hip as we went along this roller coaster type ride. Then all of a sudden, the bus driver slammed on his brakes and we came to a startling halt. The chickens went flying under the seats toward the front of the bus. I lifted my legs to give them a straight shot to the front. The goat toppled over and we all were jolted away from our seats. As I peered around my seat to see what the problem was, I saw a large gray elephant in the middle of the road. Now I am thinking, go around! Blow your horn! Do something to move this humongous beast off the road. The other passengers didn't appear to be alarmed at all. They sat quietly and waited. I became a little uncomfortable and annoyed, but I soon settled into a more calming state seeing that no one else was complaining or even seemed to care.

Don't let this disturb your peace I thought to myself. I am enjoying this adventure and I will wait with the others and be calm. Deciding to have a positive attitude makes a tremendous difference in how you feel and respond to the rest of your day.

Actually, this was the perfect opportunity for me to start up a conversation with the Chief. Of course, my first questions were "What's the problem with the elephant? Why hasn't he moved yet? Can't the driver get the elephant to move off the road?"

The Chief's response was, "You don't move an elephant; it will move when it is ready." I think he was saying to himself, "Foreigners- always in a hurry."

While we waited, the Chief and I began to chat. He spoke English fairly well and I got to learn more about the Massai tribe, their culture and traditions and he learned more about people of color in America as seen through my eyes. I enjoyed sharing information with him so much, that I felt like I should give him something, some small representation of our meeting. As we sat silently for a short while, my mind drifted as I peered out the bus window. I wondered what it would be like to live here. As I quickly snapped out of those thoughts, the Chief extended the palm of his hand toward me with one of his earrings resting within. I think our thought connected right at that moment. I quickly took off one of my earrings to do the same, I extended my hand palm up and we exchanged earrings. I gave him one of mine, a large silver dangling hoop earring, and he gave me his, a large beaded red, blue and yellow circular earring. It was a good feeling and sort of a spiritual exchange. It was from that day forth that I have been known to wear one earring, or two different earrings. It is my trademark.

The elephant finally moved and we continued on our journey. About an hour into our trip, the bus stopped again. I found out it was a bathroom stop, but where was the bathroom? One by one, I watched the women file off the bus and into the bushes, about 30 yards from the bus. I quickly got up from my seat and followed the women, remembering this is just one of many experiences, despite my hesitation, I stayed positive. Each woman positioned herself about two or three yards from the other, squatting to do their business. I watched them out of the corner of my eye, trying hard not to be conspicuous. I watched as they squatted very low; I did the same. I had some tissues in my pocket so I used them to clean myself when I was finished.

That was my first time learning how to do, what I found out later to be called the Vietnamese Squat. This was known amongst our armed service men and women, who had to acquire this knowledge in order to survive in the jungles of Vietnam. The positioning for this athletic feat was a deep knee bend with the legs straddled about three feet apart. This positioning is absolutely necessary for a clean break. An excellent piece of detailed information, particularly if you are ever find yourself in a similar situation. I, now, had experienced a part of this culture. It was different from anything I was use to, but it went with the territory, and I was pioneering my way into unchartered territory. I actually felt quite good about it.

I learned a lot about the people and culture from the Chief that day, and I learned a great deal about myself. As we continued on, I was sure I was about to learn more.

As we entered the city of Dar Es Salaam, Tanzania, which was our final destination, we stopped again for another bathroom break. This time, there was an actual restroom facility. I followed the women in and stopped dead in my tracks. There, all around the floor, were piles of feces. I looked up and there were about five or six stalls, but there was very little room to maneuver strategically to any of them. At that point, I realized, it was probably worse in those stalls, I would just have to delay the obvious and restrain myself from any further movement into that bathroom. Any pressure I might have felt had completely vanished from my body's innate reflexes. I returned to the bus.

I was in Dar Es Salaam now and the Hotel could not be that far away. Once again, I was determined that witnessing this, was not going to ruin my trip or cause me to make any snap judgments about the people, the culture, or the town.

I was going to put it out of my mind and continue with my adventure with a positive outlook.

Keeping my experience in mind, you should remember to bring with you on any trip, disinfecting wipes, disposable seat covers, tissues and hand cleansers. Disposable seat covers are just as important to pack as your underwear. You can catch diarrhea, intestinal bugs and hepatitis from toilet seats.

When toilets are flushed, a fine mist of water that could contain fecal bacteria can disperse on the toilet seats and flush handles, as well as being airborne. This doubles you chances of contracting fecal bacteria. These bacteria can be contagious. Make sure you **stand** before flushing.

(Source: Dr. C. Gerba, University of Arizona)

And so, I state once again, when traveling and encountering some environmental abnormalities, putrid smells or unsightly conditions or circumstances, and you will, just go with the flow; keep moving and don't let a potential negative experience turn you off or cause you to miss an important, cultural, or educational event.

Stay positive, stay focused, be thankful and be grateful for all experiences, for they teach us about the world and our relationship to it. You will come to understand the relativity of all things, the living spirit and beauty that manifest from a simple breeze, the smallest pebble or a shared smile from someone you just met. With eyes open, and with eyes closed, view the world from your inner spirit and much will be revealed to you.

# CHAPTER 3

⌀

# THE IMMUNE SYSTEM

The key to optimal health is found in your immune system. You have probably noticed that some people seem to be sick all the time and experience every ailment in the book, while others seem to do well through the year and especially during the winter season without a problem. This is due to the strength of one's immune system. Those, who do not get sick when flu or cold season hits have a stronger immune system. For example:"You don't catch a cold, a cold catches you". By this I mean that if your immune system is weak, you are more susceptible to colds. Colds are a bodily defense reaction to a toxic polluted body system and or an imbalance of minerals and vitamins. A disease or toxic body has very little defense against viruses and bacteria. An unhealthy, toxic body is the perfect environment for viruses and bacteria to replicate and run havoc through your body.

The mucous discharge from a cold is the body's mechanism to rid itself of waste that could not be disposed of or eliminated through the bowels, micturition or perspiration. Diseases are waiting to manifest in your body when your immune system is compromised. With a weakened immune system, you can contract, not only a cold, but sore throats, headaches, stomach problems, diarrhea, body aches, pains and much more.

With a strong immune system, you will be a fortress against the forces of disease. You will not be susceptible to the environmental, air borne, or bacterial forces that are lurking all the time.

Further, the role of the immune system is to protect the body from viruses, bacteria, fungi, and parasites that we are exposed to on a daily basis. Our bodies are under attack every day from toxins we breathe, the "fast foods" we eat and sometimes the liquids we drink.

However, our bodies are so wonderfully made that they can attack any foreign substance and bring us back to optimal health. If we treat our bodies properly, through exercise, proper nutrition, consumption of good water, consistent sleeping habits, the elimination of toxins, and positive thinking, we can keep our bodies virtually disease free.

In the summer of 2005, my husband, daughter and I took a trip to Egypt with a group of adults and children, about 200 of us in all. The first two days went well as we visited the various tombs, temples and Pyramids. We dined at the hotel for breakfast at 5:00am, and then began our day of tours so we might return to the hotel by noon because of the intense heat that comes with each day in that part of the world, especially during the months of June through September. We bought plenty of bottled drinking water, and, of course I had my bag of herbs and supplements. We stayed in the hotel during the hottest part of the day, while we prepared for the evening dinner, festivities and further excursions.

On the third day, we had a special dinner and entertainment outside on a small island on the banks of the Nile River. We were all required to wear white as this was also going to be a ceremonious affair, and a ceremony for renewing wedding vows. Like several other married couples my husband and I had planned to renew our marriage vows by partaking in this traditional African ceremony.

We all gathered at the dock near the hotel as we awaited our transport to the Egyptian Island. We soon heard the sound of drumming in the distance and saw a myriad of small tiki-like lights approaching. It was a magnificent sight - like floating stars against a black velvety sky. A fleet of eight boats were approaching as the drumming and music became louder. As they approached, we were greeted by the indigenous Nubians of the Nile, dressed in their traditional garb and playing their traditional music. We began to embark, about 30 passengers to a boat. We were entertained with music and drumming as we cruised up the Nile.

When we reached our destination, we exited the boat and walked about fifty yards up a slanted hilltop covered with Golden African sand. We took our shoes off to feel the sensation of that golden sand between our toes.

We climbed a set of stairs to reach the hilltop where a buffet dinner was colorfully displayed. Lamb and chicken were roasting on skewers and fish was offered as an option for vegetarians. There were about 20 round, low tables, about two and a half feet from the ground, decorated with tablecloths that displayed the rich hues by which African cloth is so often represented. Large African decorated pillows surrounded each table. After basking in the breath taking scenery, everyone moved toward the buffet tables to fill our plates with the various dishes that were prepared just for us. We were all ready to dine in the style of our ancestors. While eating, I noticed that all the food was uncovered and wondered how long the food had been exposed to the atmospheric elements i.e., the dessert heat. Even at night, it was hot- the perfect environment for bacteria to grow.

The uncovered food in the intense heat was my first clue that this food might cause a problem. I immediately pulled out my healing bag, and gave a large dose of collidial silver to my husband, daughter and myself. I knew then that our health would be protected against whatever bacteria was lurking in our food. We continued to fill our plates with the delicious food then sat on the big comfy pillows to dine and watch the entertainment.

The next morning, we prepared for our next excursion to Aswan.

I noticed there were only a few people standing in the lobby. As I inquired as to where everyone was, the answer came back that they were all sick. Some had stomach pain, while others experienced headaches. But one thing they all had in common was diarrhea. Well, this was no surprise to me. I knew it was the buffet dinner, which looked so appetizing, but was dangerously filled with bacteria as it sat in the heat of an open forum. And for how long, we didn't know. Later that same day, when the few of us who were able to travel returned from our morning excursion, I heard a knock on my hotel room door. It was several of the travelers asking me if I had anything that could give them relief from their symptoms. Because I was well prepared, I gave each one something from my bag that related to their individual complaint. About an hour later, more knocks were heard at my door. The word had spread- that the good doctor had a cure for whatever ailed them. Soon, I had about 20 people and counting, who needed my help. Luckily, I was able to ration out what I had and helped all in need. We still had another nine days to go, and I didn't want to be left without enough for me and my family, so I informed all travelers to be very careful of what they consume for the rest of the trip.

This is just one story out of many, as I travel the world with my bag of cures. You too can prepare your bag, and in the next chapter I will explain how you too can travel and never get sick.

The strength of the immune system is the most critical factor that separates the sick from the healthy. The cells and chemicals in the body protect your entire being, guard your intestinal tract and mucous membranes, and also monitors your bloodstream. Armed with this information, it is now time to change your thinking on how to stay well and live a healthy and fulfilled life so that you may travel the world and never be sick again.

A poor diet or too much stress also weakens the immune system, leaving the body susceptible to illness. Toxins, both externally and internally can build up in the body leaving you weak, tired, exhausted and fatigued. External toxins include, pesticides, insecticides environmental pollutants, household products, heavy metal absorption such as mercury from teeth fillings, lead from pipes in older homes, and aluminum. Internal toxins are those made in the body by improper digestion of food leading to an impacted colon. Medicines (including over-the-counter drugs), chemically engineered foods, dyes (including hair dye and chemicals added to foods such as preservatives), processed and packaged food, and foods that lack nutrients. Negative thinking and emotional stresses, such as fear, jealousy, anxiety, and depression have a tremendous negative impact on the immune system. If the body gets bombarded with more toxins than it can eliminate, then waste products will show up in your liver, kidney, sweat glands and lymphatic system. You may even develop acne and boils on your face and skin. Constipation, gastric problems, dry skin and hair, body odor, joint pain, excretions from the nose and eyes, dry mouth, flu-like symptoms, skin rashes or other serious health conditions are other symptoms of a toxic body.

Good nutrition, adequate rest, positive thinking, exercise and low stress levels are imperative for maintaining a strong and healthy immune system.

My parents, who were wholistic advocates, (wholistic meaning body mind and spirit as one) This wholistic concept is not a new concept by any means. As far back as Ancient Egypt, the Egyptians knew the body must be in balance with itself and that all three, body, mind and spirit must be in harmony in order to reach perfect health and homeostasis.

This wholistic concept was taught by my father to his family.

He taught us how to eat healthy, what to eat, how to eliminate and how to take care of our bodies and minds. We ate fruits that were only in season, we chewed our milk because it was considered a food. We ate steamed vegetables. We ate only free-roaming chickens and turkeys and not those raised in cages. On Fridays we ate fish. Soda and carbonated drinks were not consumed in our household, and diary was eaten sparingly. Sweets were allowed occasionally and only if my parents bought them from the health food store. Ice cream and cake were only served at birthday parties. No bleached white flour products, including rice and white sugar, were ever used in our home, and our wheat bread was delivered by the Dugan's bread truck once a week.

(Just a side note, bleached flour causes constipation, because it has no fiber or digestible roughage). With a diet like this, we very rarely got sick. However, when my parents detected the slightest sign of sickness or a cold, cleaning the colon was the first order of the day. Enemas always worked for us, and to this day it is the very first thing I do for myself, and recommend for my family and patients. Thanks Mom and Dad, it continues to be one of the most valuable treatments for sickness and disease.

The mind, another aspect important to the immune system, is a terrible thing to waste, and my mother knew this extremely well. She taught us powerful bible verses and repeated them often so we would not forget. She taught the power of positive thinking as she had learned from Dr. Norman Vincent Peale.

Exercising the body, is also as important as exercising the mind. We didn't have computers while I was growing up, so we spent hours playing outside the house and were glad to do so. This is how we received our exercise, we ran, rode our bikes, played tag, hop scotch and hide and seek, ice skating, went bowling and played volley ball. We were very active children.

Overwork, stress, poor diet, sedentary habits and insufficient sleep can consume the vitality of the immune system. If your immune system is compromised in any of these ways, you are susceptible to sickness. Therefore-when you are sick and begin to recover, you should not travel abroad if at all possible, for at least a week or two, especially to third world countries. Your body still needs time to recuperate and build your immune system back into a healthy state.

The number one cause of immune deficiency and weakness is micronutrient starvation, a shortage of vitamins, minerals and phytochemicals in the body which are protective plant based substances. Supplements are organic foods which can give our bodies what we need on a daily basis. These nutrients are supposed to be abundant in fresh fruits and vegetables. All too often the fruits and vegetables we buy in the supermarkets are deficient in the micronutrients that are required daily. They are also full of pesticides, toxins and insecticides. Much of our food today is genetically engineered, packaged and processed and is deficient of vitamins and minerals. Fast foods are full of toxins and made to fill you out, not fill you in with nutrition. Seventy five percent (75%) of Americans are not consuming the daily requirements needed for protection against disease and illness. Even if you think you are consuming lots of veggies and fruits, the bad news is that farmers are not putting back the nutrients into the soil once harvested. It becomes a matter of economics, and not nutrition and health. In most instances we are consuming foods that is denatured or lack the initial vitamin content they claims to have. It's not totally the farmers' fault as they are regulated by the government and they have to find ways to cut their costs. This means that the powers that be are not concerned about us and our health, but are concerned with profit. With this being said, we must take responsibility for our own health and supply our bodies with the missing elements. And if we are listening, trusting and paying attention to our bodies, they will always let us know what is missing. We will crave it. For example, when you crave a specific type of food, i.e. sugary, salty, meat, salad, green vegetables, ice cream, etc., your body is telling you that you are missing something that your body needs or wants. You may interpret it as something you have a taste for, but what the body is really saying is, "I am missing a nutrient and I need it now in order to continue to function the way I am supposed to". So what you do is fulfill that need. This is generally the case unless you have a visceral malfunction or disease, such as diabetes, liver or kidney problems. Therefore craving that ice cream doesn't mean you need just that, it means the body is telling you it needs a specific nutrient. Your mind is interpreting it as "I need sugar". When your body is getting the proper nutrients, it will crave less of the sugar and salty foods.

To maximize your intake of much needed nutrients, eat organic if you can, shop at local farmers markets, and eat for color. That means, choose deep colored fruits and vegetables.

These are filled with natural disease fighting phytochemicals, such as carotenoids and flavonoids. Eat raw fruit, and drink fresh fruit juices. Use almond butter, almond milk, rice milk, soy, and or vegetable protein drinks. Eat wheat, oats grains and fiber daily. All meats should be baked or broiled and without added oil.

# CHAPTER 4

⌒∿⌒

# COLON HEALTH

Growing up, one of our most feared pieces of wholistic equipment was the dreaded enema bag. If you dared to say you were sick, out came the RED bag of terror. It was a red rubber bag about 14 inches long and 12 inches wide, with a small hose attached to the bottom end of the bag, which then allowed for another small bulb-like attachment with several small holes at the end to be inserted into the rectum. At the top of the bag was an opening large enough to pour one quart of warm water into it. This was used for the infusion. The warm water activated the motility of the colon, which would help to eliminate feces that had become plaqued (almost cement like) to the sides of the colon. This plaquing actually causes most of the discomfort, such as constipation, gas and internal toxins. This plaque generally has been stuck on the sides of the colon for days, weeks and even months, causing not only discomfort, but can cause sickness and diseases such as colon cancer, diverticulitis, appendicitis, spastic colon and even Colitis. My father's belief, as is mine today, was that the seat of disease lies in the colon. Clean the colon first, which helps to rid your body of the harmful toxins that are the culprit for many diseases and pain.

This proved to be true in every case for me and my siblings. We stayed well throughout our childhood, mainly because of that red bag, and a proper diet without processed foods. My patients today enjoy a healthier and fulfilling life because they keep their colons clean and follow a program of healthy foods, exercise and positive thinking. These practices are absolutely essential to your optimal health.

I attended a conference in Jamaica in the early fall of 2001. My first evening at a beautiful beach hotel, a traditional Jamaican buffet by the pool was prepared for the participants. It was a grand lay out of curry goat, jerk chicken, peas and rice, plantains, callaloo, ackee and more. I filled my plate, ate all I could and finished off the meal with a Jamaican desert. Later that night my gastro-intestinal track was screaming for help. I had ingested some foreign material that didn't agree with my system. Stomach pain and cramps had me doubled over in the bed. Luckily, I had a bottle of colon cleanser with me in my herbal bag. In pain, I managed to gather together the capsules with a large bottle of water. I took 3 and lied down on the bed, trying to find a comfortable position so that I might get some sleep. The next morning, I was still very sick with stomach pains and cramps. In between my trips to the bathroom I took another 3 capsules of the colon cleanser. I wasn't surprised that I was not hungry, because I knew my body had to rid itself of the bacteria, so putting more food in would just create a food source or more energy for the bacteria to stay alive. It was an absolute necessity to cleanse first. I drank more water then went back to bed. Later that afternoon, I felt a little better. I stayed in my room so I could be close to the bathroom. I took 3 more capsules and drank more water. I went back to bed. By the third day, I was up, feeling stronger and had finally eliminated the bacteria that ran havoc through my system. I showered, got dressed and joined the others. I was very careful with my food selections on the remainder of the trip.

# CHAPTER 5

⌒𝓂⌒

# PREPARATION

Preparation. Get your immune system in order before you travel, and if by chance you do become sick before your date of departure, I have a few tips for you as well.

Now we are ready for a step- by- step gathering of all you need.

Carotenoids are among the most widespread pigments in the natural world. They play a large role in healing, and their colorful appearance is attractive to the eye and the palate. They are represented in foods like red peppers, tomatoes, paprika and salmon.* Add these type of carotenoids to your daily diet.

Flavonoids are strong antioxidants found in plants that act as hormone blockers in the body where excess hormones could cause cancer, such as breast cancer. They are represented by foods such as cranberries, apples, peanuts, chocolate (surprise!) and onions.* Flavonoids are a wonderful addition to anyone's normal diet. Because these act as antioxidants, eat plenty to help strengthen your immune system. Regular exercise, proper diet, and chiropractic adjustments that help keep your body in alignment will help in boosting your immune system. Positive thinking we well know, also contributes to a healthy and energized immune system. Learn to speak positive and uplifting words to yourself and others; put positive and healthy, healing concepts into your everyday life. Be aware of how you feel each day. Monitor your feelings, emotions and stress levels, learn to be your own doctor. Then… "Doctor Heal Thy Self".

The following are further steps you can follow to boost your immune system and to stay healthy before embarking on your trip.

Step 1: In your carry on bag, pack all medications you are currently taking. Make sure you have more than enough.

Step 2: Whether you have allergies or not, be sure to pack some type of over the counter allergy medication. Allergies are generally a failure to breakdown a particular type of food or nutrient. A Whole foods diet before your trip such as organic fruits and vegetables will decrease episodes. Also avoid junk foods.

Step 3:  Purchase the following items from your local health food store or pharmacy.

(+) 1 bottle of chewable Vitamin C tablets 500mil.

(++) 1 to 2 bottles of Colloidal Silver. 1oz (depending how long you will be away)

(+) 1 bottle of Charcoal tablets (90 tabs)

(+) 1 to 2 bottles of Odorless garlic oil capsules (not pills) 60 capsules

1 Bottle of liquid Capsicum 1 oz.

(++) 1 Bottle/bag or box of Colon Cleansers (no laxatives)

1 small bottle of peppermint oil

1 bottle Vitamin High B complex or Vitamin B12 sublingual (means under the tongue)

1 small bottle of Melatonin

1 small bottle of aspirin

(+) Disinfecting wipes

(+) Hand Cleanser

Continue to take your daily vitamins. If you are not taking a daily vitamin, you should purchase a bottle. If you have any other supplements, take them with you as well. Take supplements that feed the cells oxygen like chlorophyll or Vita Mineral Greens. It is not a deal breaker if you don't purchase all the recommended items but it is a must that you take all the checked (+) ones.

Step 4:  Eat plenty of foods rich in vitamins. Eat seasonal fruits and vegetables. Beets, red grapes, apricots, sesame seeds, nuts, blueberries, cherries, carrots, green leafy vegetables, especially spinach, kale and mustard greens, (steamed not boiled), watermelon, cantaloupes, pomegranates, papaya, oranges, grapefruits and lemons. Be sure not to mix melons with any other fruit, they should be eaten separately. Again, if you are eating meat, it should be baked or broiled with no extra oil.

## VITAMIN C*

The Vitamin nomenclature comes from the word vital, meaning "vital to life".

The difference between vitamins and minerals, is that vitamins energize the body. While minerals stabilize the body. All vitamins are enzymes and all enzymes are vitamins. You can take a handful of Vitamin "C" with you each day. Take them periodically throughout the day. Your body will only absorb about 300 milligrams at any one time and will expel what it doesn't use when you urinate. Don't be alarmed if your Urine is a dark yellow color, this is due to the Vitamin C eliminating what the body doesn't need or use.

## COLLOIDAL SILVER*

Colloidal Silver has been known as a remarkably effective natural antibiotic for centuries. Silver's innate anti-microbial effect was actually common knowledge among doctors for over 90 years. This product will be in a liquid form, clear to a very slight yellow tint. It comes with a dropper for your convenience.

Put one dropper in each of the bottled drinking water you consume each day. Therefore if you drink 3 to 6 bottles of water each day, then each bottle will have one dropper full of Silver Colloidal.

You may read more about this wonderful natural antibiotic in the research done by Dr. Robert O. Becker, one of many doctors who have researched this product.

## CHARCOAL TABLETS*

Charcoal is the miracle of absorption. It is used to treat stomach pain caused by gas, diarrhea and indigestion, and has been used in severe food poisoning. At the first sign of stomach discomfort follow the directions on the bottle for the dosage, or take exactly as prescribed by your Health Care Professional. DO NOT take charcoal with any other medicines. Take the tablets either 2 hours before or 1 hour after medications. DO NOT use charcoal if you are allergic to charcoal or if you have liver or kidney disease. And always consult your natural health care professional or herbal doctor.

## GARLIC OIL* (the wonder drug)

If the name wonder drug can be applied to any healing herb, garlic is the one. It is the world's second oldest medicine and still remains the best.

Garlic was prescribed by Hippocrates as a natural cure-all in his ancient manuscripts. Today, it is known also as a cure all because of its high concentration of sulfur compounds. Garlic is shown to have anti-microbial activity against many disease causing organisms. Taken everyday helps in the overall well being of the systems of the body.

Garlic is known to lower blood pressure by 20-30mm. And when you travel to extremely hot climates it is essential to take this wonder oil with you. Garlic is also known to lower cholesterol, has germ killing compounds, fights off bacterial, viral, urinary and fungal infections, and is known to fight urinary tract infections as well. It can also act as a decongestant and expectorant. So when you have a cold, garlic is the natural cure. Garlic is also known to ward off mosquitoes and other bugs. Each day take 6 to 8 oil capsules. They are very small, so you can take them all at one time. This can help in prevention of bacterial infections, the prevention of colds and warding off mosquitoes as well. Increase to 8-10 capsules if you are in an area heavily infected with mosquitoes. This treatment was very effective for me when traveling through the Amazon, Laos and parts of Brazil.

*If you have a clotting disorder, consult your health care provider before taking the medicinal amount. For otherwise healthy, non pregnant non-nursing adults who do not have a clotting disorders, garlic is considered safe even in large amounts. Garlic is known to have a strong odor. If you are worried about the smell or offending others, you can eliminate garlic breath by trying traditional herbal breath fresheners, such as parsley, fennel or fenugreek, or a standard breath freshener or mint if you prefer.

This reminds me of a great story about garlic. In April of 2007, my travel partners and I made a trip to the Brazil. Our plan was to spend time in Rio De Janeiro, then to Bahia then off to the Amazon. I had casually read up on the Amazon rainforest and the surrounding areas of Brazil. I read about the plant life, wild life and the river. But nothing could compare with observing it with your own eyes.

The Negro River was particularly of interest to me and I'll tell you why. The Negro River is almost two thousand miles long, and its waters are totally black. This river claims to contain the richest minerals anywhere in the world. The waters that flow down from the Andes into the Negro River contain organic material from the rain forest, adding to the minerals already present, rendering the waters black. It was my first time ever seeing black waters. It was mysterious, awesome and haunting all at once. We traveled down the river with our guide in a medium sized motor powered boat that accommodated all ten of us.

The great Mother Earth and its entire splendor are displayed with GOD's Omni- present paint brush on all sides of the banks. The wild life and vegetation there were displayed in all the splendid colors. The deep emerald green palm leaves spread out like a china fan. The feathers of the macaws were like an array of illuminated rainbows. The colors of flora and fauna were like being in a marvelous botanical garden. You can feel the spirit of the jungle breathing through the powerful and enormous Liana trees. The roots of these trees were entwined with each other as well as coiled around its massive trunk. Many limbs and roots were serpent like as they tightly wrapped themselves around and around like the stripes of a candy cane. The guide maneuvered our boat toward the bank. As we exited the boat we could see a definite dirt trail. It was obvious this trail was well traveled and a regular part of our tour into the rainforest. The feeling of being protected and incase by these giant trees was exhilarating. Looking straight up between the Liana trees gave impulses of light. Leaves of all sizes and shapes seem to compete for the sunlight, yet they blocked out most of the sun, but still leaving us in a tropical cover of shade.

We stopped temporarily to listen to the sounds of the forest that stimulated our sense of hearing and peaked our curiosity about the creatures that actually live in this jungle. I gave thanks to the spirit and energy of Mother Nature.

We continued on. The terrain was just slightly elevated with a moderate downward progression, a course easily maneuvered even for those who were not so physically fit. I stayed close to our guide to hear everything he had to share about the environment.

It was extremely hot as the temperature had metamorphosed into a sweltering dense atmosphere, which was evident by our perspiration and viscous like skin. As our guide took us further into the jungle, my husband and I began to notice how uneasy the other travelers were becoming as they swatted off the numerous mosquitoes that seem to be ensuing us. They began spraying more "Bug Off" on their clothing, but it did very little to keep away the mosquitoes. My husband and I weren't bothered with them at all. I contribute this to the fact that we had been taking 10 odorless garlic oil capsules a day. These capsules not only helped kept us healthy, but also aided in the protection against those mosquitoes.

CAPSICUM (Cayenne pepper)*
Capsicum is a phytochemical used for many conditions, such as raising your metabolic rate (the rate at which your body burns fat while at resting). It will lower LDL's, (bad cholesterol), but raises the HDL's (the good cholesterol), according to studies done in the United States and India.

Capsicum is known to stop heart attacks, heartburn, stomach aches, ulcers and irritable bowel syndrome. I suggest taking this with you. It will be to your advantage if you experience circulation or heart problems. Capsicum will activate the heart in case of heart burn or symptoms that may appear as a heart attack. Avoid taking aspirin or any blood thinners if you are going to use this product. It is also NOT recommended for any gastro-esophageal reflex diseases or to be used with asthma medications. For an infusion and to aid in digestion and possible reduction in the risk for heart disease use:    ¼ to ½ teaspoon per cup of boiling water after meals. For external application to help treat pain:Mix ¼ to ½ teaspoon per cup of warm vegetable oil, or Castrol and rub into the affected area. Do not give to children under the age of 2. For younger children, start with a smaller amount and use more if necessary. People over 65 often have a decrease in taste buds and skin sensitivity, and may require more than younger adults.

If you experience any heart-related symptoms and cannot reach your doctor, it is suggested that you take one dropper full for emergencies. Then immediately seek professional help.

**Before taking this product or any other product suggested here, be sure to consult with your health care professional.**

COLON CLEANSERS*
This is a big one. When we travel we tend to become constipated because of the change in eating habits as well as any time change from one country to the next. This will impact you depending on where your destination may be. You absolutely must ELIMINATE, EVACUATE, and cleanse the colon from what you eat on a daily

basis at least two to three times a day, depending on how many meals you have consumed. One to two hours after consumption, you should be evacuating. Find a good colon cleanser in your local health food store. You want to have something gentle, working with your regular body rhythm and NOT something where you require a bathroom nearby at all times.

Colon cleansers should be taken at the end of your day. It generally takes anywhere from 6 to 10 hours to work, depending on your system. If you take it at night, two to three hours before bedtime, you should have excellent results by morning and would not need to worry about the rest of the day. If you haven't moved your bowels by morning however, take precautions throughout the day. It may take a little longer for you, because your system is specific in its function. So you may want to stay near a bathroom. Colon cleansers will not react the same as laxatives, so you should not experience the "got to go" feeling during the day. You may have to go during the day, but most trips and tours around the world will have bathroom stops. So, don't worry. You may not have to take colon cleansers everyday. You may only require them when you have not evacuated on any day you feel sluggish. You should also take a colon cleanser if you become ill, or experience chills or fever. Removing bacteria from the body through the colon is required to return to optimal health. Your stools should be floating and rust to brown in color. If they appear green or black or any other color **continue** using the cleansers until your stool has returned to its normal color. Discoloration and odor, simply means your·body is trying to rid itself of foreign material toxins and bacteria.

## PEPPERMINT OIL*

Peppermint contains menthol that is highly recommended as a digestive aid, decongestant, and anesthetic. It is also known for its germicidal properties. Peppermint has its roots and uses far back as ancient Egypt. Peppermint was mentioned in the world's oldest medical text, the *Ebers Papyrus*. It was an ancient custom of ending a feast with a sprig of mint to soothe the stomach. We have all had our experiences with this menthol through the use of the after dinner mint, its use in morning sickness in pregnant woman, upset stomachs, it is a main ingredient in Vicks Vapor Rub and a myriad of other products. Science has lent support to this age old practice: best known for its uses in flavors such as candies, gum, toothpastes and mouthwashes. Peppermint oil is good to travel with in that inhaling it will open up the sinuses and allow free breathing. If you feel your breathing being compromised when traveling due to atmospheric changes, take a small inhalation from the bottle, or put a dash of the oil below your nostrils, which will open your sinuses. You can also put a small drop or two on the back of your wrist, lick off with the tongue, which will also help to open the sinuses and soothe any stomach irritation. The menthol vapors help relieve nasal, sinus and chest congestion. Peppermint is a Food and Drug Administration –approved remedy for the common cold, primarily for its decongestive action.

## B COMPLEX*

The B vitamins are excellent for your nerves and overall health. It becomes a necessity if you are suffering from certain deficiencies. If you are a nervous person and have general stress and anxiety of travel, you might want to pick up a bottle of B vitamins or sublingual B12. Vitamin B Complex contains B1, B2, B3, B4,

B6, B12 and B13. B complex is highly suggested to people with digestive problems, loss of appetite, constipation, muscle weakness, nervousness, insomnia, headaches, fatigue, and mental depression. Vitamin B complex increases the use of body proteins, aids in digestion, helps to prevent fluid retention, increase circulation and assist in the assimilation and metabolism of proteins and fats. It is particularly useful in the nervous system and mental cognition in that it helps the body to use oxygen.

MELATONIN*

Frequent flyers have testified to the wonderful results they have received from using this supplement especially if the flight is over 8 to 10 hours, or if you are leaving on a "Red Eye" flight. It has reduced their jet lag and re-programmed their body's clock so they may feel refreshed upon arrival. This may be the supplement for you to regain your alertness and vitality and to enjoy the day you arrive. If you are traveling into another time zone, purchase a small bottle of Melatonin and follow the directions on the label. An example is that you should take one or two capsules 2 hours before you would normally go to sleep (which will probably be on the plane). This will help you to fall asleep naturally, then awake refreshed. Be aware of the time you are to arrive at your destination. If your arrival is at night, you should wait until you have reached your hotel before taking this supplement. If your arrival is in the daytime and you left home in the daytime, then you should take the Melatonin capsules at your normal bedtime.

You must check your schedule of activities before deciding when to take the capsules. You will have a normal sleep without any drowsiness or after effects. Melatonin is a natural product that works well with your body's natural sleep mechanism.

ASPIRIN/ADVIL/ALEVE*

Have a pain reliever, such as aspirin, advil or aleve on hand just in case. But take only if absolutely necessary. The less allopathic drugs in the system, the better for you and your overall health. If you are experiencing headaches, find a quiet place, close your eyes and breathe deeply for a few minutes, relax. If your headache is stress related, this exercise will help.

*(Source: M. Castleman, Healing Herbs)

WATER

Drinking water every day is a must, just as you do normally when not traveling. But please BEWARE. Most countries sell bottled water and you should always buy bottled water, preferably the ones with a 3, 5 or 7 rating. You can find this rating at the bottom of the bottle in the small triangle. These bottled waters are rated on their leaching factor (toxins from the plastic bottle that leach or infuse themselves into the water). This is another reason why you will put the Colloidal Silver directly into your bottle of water. Drink plenty of water while traveling, especially now that you know what to do. Water helps to flush your system and will keep you hydrated. REMEMBER; DO NOT BRUSH YOUR TEETH WITH FACET WATER. Use your bottle water to cleanse your teeth.

Avoid ice if at all possible. If not, make sure you have your colloidal silver with you to counteract any adverse side effects.

If you have any other supplements that you are taking, be sure to bring them. Most supplements and herbs have no negative effect in combination with allopathic drugs, but be sure to consult with a natural health care practitioner before your trip.

## FOODS TO EAT AND FOODS TO AVOID

My travels throughout Asia were one of my most memorable events. The reason is that the climate there is the most conducive for growing the most fabulous, colorful and delicious fruits and vegetables.

I remember my trip to Thailand, a country of good food, good people, good weather, good shopping and fantastic massages. You must be careful, however when eating Thai food from floating markets or street vendors. My daughter and I visited the famous "Floating Market" located outside of Bangkok with a tour group. We witnessed for ourselves the numerous amount of people who took ill that day because of food consumed from such a venue.

As the tour bus reached the market, we exited the bus and headed toward the wooden, fish tail type boats. We boarded the boats eight at a time and sped along the waterway powered by a small but powerful motor. We passed the homes of the rural Thai's as we watched them in their daily routine. Some were fishing, and cooking while others washed clothes. Children splashed about in the water while others just relaxed trying to cool off from the very hot temperatures of a normal Thai day.

We continued up the fairly narrow waterway, passing other fishtail boats, other travelers and the awesome greenery and amazing colorful plants, flowers and trees. Along the way, vendors were serving all types of cooked foods and fresh fruits. They were so colorful, titillating, and a delight for the five senses especially that of smell and sight. The people were friendly, happy and anxious to see a group of tourists. We stopped along the way to look at each large stir fry pan and tried to identify what the dish might be. My daughter and I took pictures of many of the dishes and jotted down the name of each. Luckily, we had a tour guide with us who helped us in the pronunciation of many of the dishes, which dishes we could sample and the cautions we should take.

Most of the food was totally unrecognizable to anything American with which we are familiar. But, it looked and smelled wonderful. Naturally, the very adventurous (and not so smart) tourists decided they would experience small samplings of a few of the dishes, despite the tour guide's warning. They said they felt fine and the food was delicious. We continued on to the floating market. Needless to say, that evening, many of them were ill.

Eat fruit that has a natural cover or protection such as bananas, cucumbers, apples and indigenous fruits. Many of the indigenous fruits are very tasty as well as colorful, such as jack fruit (a sweet yellow fruit covered with a thick skin) pineapples, dragon fruit, mangoes, papaya, strawberries, coconut, gooseberry (a small yellow berry used in deserts and jams), guava, jujube (a similar taste to the apple, called Thai apple) Litchee ( a sweet, juicy fruit inside a hard, red peel,) mangosteen (dark purple peel with sweet, white fruit inside) and many others. This is the venue with which you can definitely experiment. The temperature in Thailand is exceptionally conducive for growing these wonderful fruits. If you are a fruit lover, you will be in fruit heaven.

Stay away from raw fish such as sushi. Stay away from open market foods that are uncovered. Eat at recommended restaurants. There are a myriad of Thai Restaurants to choose from with the traditional Thai and International cuisine. Thai noodles are a must to try and a popular taste of Bangkok. Great coffee and deserts are among the array of tasty goods.

Make sure your food is cooked thoroughly. Parasites are just lurking to find a good host. Parasitic infections may spread through contaminated water, fruits, vegetables, grains, poultry, fish, and meat. When purchasing fruits and vegetables make sure you wash them thoroughly. Signs of infection include a runny nose, nighttime restlessness, a feeling of being bloated, tired and hungry. You may experience allergies, anemia, lethargy, fuzzy thinking, headaches and roller coaster blood sugar levels. Other symptoms may include hair loss, diarrhea, arthritis, mineral imbalances and nighttime teeth grinding. One or more symptoms may occur to a greater or lesser degree depending on the individual. These uninvited guests come in four different groups: roundworms, tapeworms, single cell protozoan and flukes. These worms exist world wide and especially in warmer climates. Pinworms are the most common in the U.S.

Tips for prevention include:

1. Cooked meats thoroughly.
2. Don't use a microwave to cook meat: microwaves do not heat foods completely.
3. Wash fruits and vegetables.
4. Always wash your hands after handling raw meat.

5. Avoid swallowing river, stream or lake water when swimming.
6. Eat high fiber foods.
   (See information in Chapter 7 for Herbal remedies to eliminate Parasites.)

Even with all the precautions you will take, there is some leeway in eating and sampling foods for the first time. If you are interested in trying something new, if you are an adventurer and globe trekker, like myself, then sample foods in very small quantities, just a taste. I have tried many different types of foods and liquids such as donkey, piranha, tentacles from a jelly fish, cobra and tiger penis liquor and all types of snake teas. Make sure you take your silver colloidal and charcoal tablets with you when sampling. Always take a dropper full of colloidal silver or a dropper in your drinking water when tasting and sampling. Be sure it is something that the indigenous people would eat or is being served in a restaurant. Use your spirit and common sense when making any decisions in a foreign country.

# CHAPTER 6

## SPIRITUAL HEALTH

### "In search of truth and knowledge of self"

We are quite aware that the body has its own health, but so does the mind and spirit. But because it is more subtle than the body, we are not so quick to detect any abnormalities which in time may develop into something more serious. The Spirit, has a health of its own. It is much more subtle than that of the mind or the body, so we are not as conscious of the deviations that take place, keeping the spirit out of balance.

We cannot deny that the body and mind are sustained by proper attention to their needs. Strangely enough, one might think by the way we live that the spirit could be expected to survive with the grossest neglect, as if it were something to be put away and ignored for awhile and then take it back at some future date when you think you might need it.

To be whole, healthy or wholistic, as we have talked about, the spirit must be addressed with the same vigor and enthusiasm as the body. Modern medicine has even discovered that optimal health is a matter which concerns the mind and spirit as well as the body. Certainly nothing is more obvious in our present condition as a lack of peace, contentment and a rich renewal of life. We have forgotten how to shut the door, enter the closet and seek inner peace and quietness. We have forgotten to restore the spirit by contemplating the SOURCE of life and from which the spirit has come. We have become spiritual insomniacs waiting for something outside ourselves to wake us up. Our waking up and listening is a sign of spiritual health and vitality.

As you travel, watch and listen, you will discover your search is mainly about your life, your spiritual health and vitality. It's your pilgrim's journey and your opportunity to ascertain who you are through people you meet, the places you go and how you respond to the stimulus all around you. It's all relative and it's your moment in time to recognize the "TRUTH".

All the great Prophets throughout their ministries, constantly and consistently emphasized the necessity of knowing the truth. And the truth is within us all, whether dormant or awake. This refers to the relationship you have with your higher power.

Each of us has the "Spirit of Truth". This is something we recognize as conscience and which will always lead us in the right direction when we obey its prompting. Its prompting many times manifest itself as that small inner voice that alerts us to a certain path of good or evil. The human spirit is not whole or healthy unless it has found that inner voice. The spirit will always be restless and discontent. Personally, I have found that traveling has given me insight into other cultures and their people, which for the past 40 years, have changed my life, my "outlook" on the world and my insight to self awareness and spirituality.

Man at his healthiest is a worshipper, listening intently to life and knowing that all he has heard and seen may be fulfilled in and through him. You are a source of vibrational energy. You are consciousness; you are creator; you are what you think. This combination of energy will lead you to all that you desire, if only you will claim it. I have included spirituality in this book, because of the myriad of energies you will encounter during your travels. By this I mean forces of nature. The forces of nature are divergent in various parts of the world. Different, in that many cultures look upon the earth and its many living organism as sacred, consequently, giving off the vibrations of the people who worship there. If you allow yourself to be unrestricted, and open to discover your innate ability, you will feel this energy. From this energy came everything into existence, visible and invisible. As you travel the world, you will come to recognize these sometimes small and subtle signs that speak to your inner spirit and subconscious. "Seek and Ye Shall Find" Knock and the Door Shall be Opened", Luke 11:9. In my words, seek it through exploration, find it with your inner guide and bring it into conscious manifestation through your Spiritual Energy, Truth and Love.

Let us be reminded of the T.S Elliot poem stated at the beginning of this book;

*We shall not cease from exploration*
*And the end of all our exploring*
*Will be to arrive where we started*
*And know the place for the time*

*"We shall not cease from exploration"* implies by our very nature, that we seek something greater than ourselves. We will constantly and consistently pursue, examine, search, investigate and explore.

Become an explorer in your search for Truth. Become a pioneer for your soul, even if you have to repeat your destination again and again. Become an adventurer of life and living.

*"At the end of all our exploring, we will arrive where we started"* Sometimes it takes more then one visit, more then one try to finally understand.

*"Knowing the place for the first time"* equates to the conscious manifestation of understanding and Truth, bringing into light that which was in darkness.

This energy is the ultimate goal in your spiritual voyage.

Whatever you think and feel yourself to be, the Creative Spirit of Life is bound to reproduce in a corresponding reaction. This is a good reason to picture yourself in your travels and in all your affairs the way you would like them to be. Positive thoughts and love will create a positive and loving experience.

# CHAPTER 7

ON YOUR RETURN

## Parasites

When you return from your wonderful adventure, there are certain things you should do as a follow up especially if you have traveled abroad. Many foods and liquids we consume in and out of the country contain parasites and worms.

You must make sure you rid yourself of any parasites and worms that you may have accumulated in your body after eating and drinking in foreign countries.

I can recall my travels in Jamaica one year, where a group of wholistic practitioners went on an excursion to Dunn River Falls. It was a beautiful hot day, as it always is in Jamaica and several of us decided to venture a little further beyond the falls. About a hundred yards away, we discovered what appeared to be a natural mud bath, and there were several people there lying in the mud and spreading it all over their bodies. Well, this seemed attractive to our group, as we all knew about the healing properties that mud possesses. The people looked relaxed and appeared to be having a good time. We all looked at each other and began to disrobe down to our bathing suits.

One jumped in, two jumped in, and as I approached to do the same, I stopped. Something within me was telling me to wait. I contemplated for a minute, then it hit me, mud, dirt, soil earth. This reminded me of the standard slip of paper given to you at customs. "Are you bringing back any wild life, plants, soil or fruits etc"? The reasons for these questions are to determine if you have come in contact with any diseased animals or plant life or returning to the States with any foreign substances that may be contaminated with bacteria, parasites, or any foreign materials not indigenous to the U.S.

I thought again, if I roll around in that mud, could I possibly contract any parasites that may bore themselves into my skin then into my blood stream? I wasn't sure, but I wasn't going to take that chance. I smiled at the others then opted out of that activity. I didn't want to alarm any of them at the time, and maybe they would have not believed me anyway.

Beware of this type of activity, unless directed by a guide or professional who will know the area and the terrain.

Knowing the area and having a guide is the smart thing to do when traveling to unfamiliar places. The Amazon was one of those places. Three of the most exciting activities I participated in, was piranha fishing in the day alligator hunting at night and swimming with the pink dolphins. The piranha fishing was uneventful for all of us except my husband Earl. He was the only one in the group who caught a piranha that day. We all watched him as he carefully baited his hook with the raw bloody meat that was given to us by the guide. He reeled in the fish that was about a foot long. The rest of us just continued to feed the piranha with no luck in catching a single one. Before Earls catch, we were all under the impression that piranha were very small, 4 to 6 inches in length and travelled in large groups, but discovered they come in a variety of sizes, over a foot long, have very hard, razor sharp teeth and mainly feed close to the river banks in the cool of the shade, hoping for something alive to fall in. Maybe they would get lucky with a small squirrel monkey. Earl took his proud catch back to the hotel restaurant, where the chef prepared it magnificently in a stew. When completed, the chef brought out his master piece directly to the table and placed it in front of my husband. The aroma was the first thing you noticed. And it was served with a presentation that Emeril would have admired. It was a mouth watering eye full. Earl shared this delight with me, and it was absolutely delicious; It was seasoned to perfection, and was complemented by the Amazon's indigenous vegetables and herbs. Earl offered the others in the group a sample, but they declined.

Part of our planned activities while we were in the Amazon, was to swim with the pink dolphins in the Negro River. As I mentioned earlier the Negro River is a river so rich in minerals. These minerals flow from the Andes Mountains in the river, rendering the color a shimmering velvety black.

The dolphins there are pink in color because they have adapted to that rich mineral environment turning their skin a light hazy pink. My travel partners were hesitant to go into the water, knowing earlier that day we went piranha fishing in that same river. Well, as the adventurous one in the group, I felt it was okay to swim in the water. After all we had a guide and he has brought many tourist to this very spot over the years and no one had never gotten eaten by piranha. I got in the water with the guide as did the daughter of one of our group members (a young adult). I found it to be quite an enjoyable experience; however the young lady was frightened by the massive bodies of the dolphins who were obviously quite friendly, because they were close and personal. She panicked for a quick minute, then began to feel more relaxed. After being in the water for about 10 minutes or so my young friend began to become accustomed to the water and to the big fish. We fed the dolphins' small fish from a white bucket that was given to us by our guide. They became quite excited but not aggressive. When we fed them the last fish, they very contently swam away, and we exited the river as well.

New activities should be a good experience for you. So don't let it stop you from having a good time. As long as you follow the directions of your guide then follow the de-worming protocol listed in this book upon your return, your experiences will be well worth the time.

One of the first things you should do on your return is to purchase a parasite cleanser such as Black Walnut Seed Extract, and Citricidal (grapefruit extract) or a para-cleanse. And now you know why.

Use 50 drops of Black Walnut Extract and 4 drops of the Grapefruit Extract, mix together in 6oz of water. Stir vigorously and drink while it is still spinning. Do this upon arising in the morning. Refill the glass with water and drink immediately. Use room temperature water, preferably, distilled or spring water. Be sure to follow these directions for at least 5 to 7 days to be sure you have cleansed the body thoroughly.

If you are using a para-cleanse, then follow the directions on the box or bottle.

Next purchase a good colon cleanser, (not a laxative). This will help to eliminate toxins and any placqued fecal matter that has accumulated on the sides of the colon from foods that you have eaten on your trip. Foods such as red meats and dairy products take a longer time for the body to digest.

For the next six days, use a "loofah" or soft to medium dry shower brush to cleanse your body in the shower, and bath. The first day you should shower, to rinse and rid the body of dead cells and toxins. Initially, a bath will only hold the dead cells and toxins in the water you sit in. Therefore a shower is recommended on the first day. You want to have running water to flush the dead cells and toxins down the drain, especially on your first day of return. On the second day, get in a hot tub (warm if you have high blood pressure) soak in 2 cups of Epsom Salt. Alternate and repeat each day between the shower and bath until the sixth day. Use the dry brush or loofah starting at the feet moving toward your head. Dry brush your face with a buff puff. When you exit from the tub or shower each day, do Peroxide therapy on your ears every other night. Peroxide is a wonderful way to cleanse all parts of the body. Purchase a bottle of 3% oral debriding Hydrogen Peroxide. Put ¼ cap in the ear while laying on your side or just tilting the head to one side. Allow the peroxide to bubble for about 5 minutes or until bubbling subsides. Drain out and dry well. Brush your teeth three times a day and floss once per day to cleanse the mouth. You can use hydrogen peroxide to brush your teeth for the maximum cleansing. You can also gargle with the solution. Do not ingest.

Personally, I have traveled to every Continent on this planet. I have followed every step outlined to you and have never gotten sick. You too, can have wonderful experiences when you plan smartly for your trips any where in the world. If you follow these simple steps and keep your immune system strong, exercise and eat healthy, you will certainly enjoy the cultural extravaganza waiting for you around the world.

So now you are ready and prepared for your trip anywhere in the world.

Make peace with your environment, appreciate nature's wisdom and you will find reward in all of nature's diversity.

# Chapter 8

CONCLUSION

As my father would say, "Life is a wonderful journey". And so it is. Let this book be your health and spiritual guide to the amazing journey that is ahead for you. Follow these simply instructions. Use your knowledge of health and wellness. Rediscover your innate ability to allow the well being of the Universe to flow steadily and unrestricted into your experience, the well being that makes up every particle, atom and cell that you are and that from which you come.

You are the creator of your own experience. Know that your positive thoughts are manifested in your desires. Create your own positive travel experience through your thought, discipline and love.

Travel well my friends.

* The products listed in this book are not approved by the FDA for treatment or cure of any illness or disease. Consult with your health care practitioner before taking any supplements or herbs. The Reverend Eugene and Mary Robinson Center for Wellness and Longevity may be contacted to answer any of your questions or concerns. Therobinsonwellnesscenter.com or 973 678-7575 or <u>drfa@verizon.net</u>

Yours, In Natural Health Care.
Dr. Fadairo Afolabi,D.C.

# About the Author

⌒⅏⌒

**Dr. Fadairo Afolabi**, known fondly by her patients as "Dr. Fa", has been a holistic Chiropractic Physician for over 16 years. She is the founder and CEO of the Rev. Eugene and Mary Robinson Center for Wellness and Longevity, which is located in East Orange, New Jersey. Dr. Fa earned her Doctorate degree from the University of Bridgeport, College of Chiropractic. She has lectured and treated patients all over the world as an advocate of chiropractic and holistic living. She has presented in Tokyo, Japan, the Amazon,Brazil, Sydney, Australia, Shanghi and Beijing, China, Egypt, Ghana and Cape Town, South Africa to name a few. She is the recipient of numerous awards and accolades, including The Chiropractor of the Year. Dr. Fa travels the world to learn more about indigenous medicine and herbal cures.